A SIMPLE GUIDE TO YOGA

BY FRANCES KEAN AND SUSAN VOORHEES

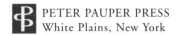

PETER PAUPER PRESS
White Plains, New York

*This book is dedicated, in humble gratitude,
to all the teachers through the ages who have diligently
transmitted the teachings of yoga.*

*Many thanks to Myra Alston
for her advice and assistance.*

Photographs:
p.4, 30-31, 48: © Don King/Image Bank
p. 18-19, 26-27, 33: © Kent Barker/Image Bank

Illustrated by Kerren Barbas
Designed by Heather Zschock

This book is not intended to replace expert medical advice.
The authors and publishers urge you to verify the appropriateness of
any procedure or exercise with your qualified health care practitioner.
The authors and publishers disclaim any liability or loss, personal or otherwise,
resulting from the procedures and information in this book.

Copyright © 2002
Peter Pauper Press, Inc.
202 Mamaroneck Avenue
White Plains, NY 10601
All rights reserved
ISBN 0-88088-416-9
Printed in China
7 6 5 4

Visit us at www.peterpauper.com

CONTENTS

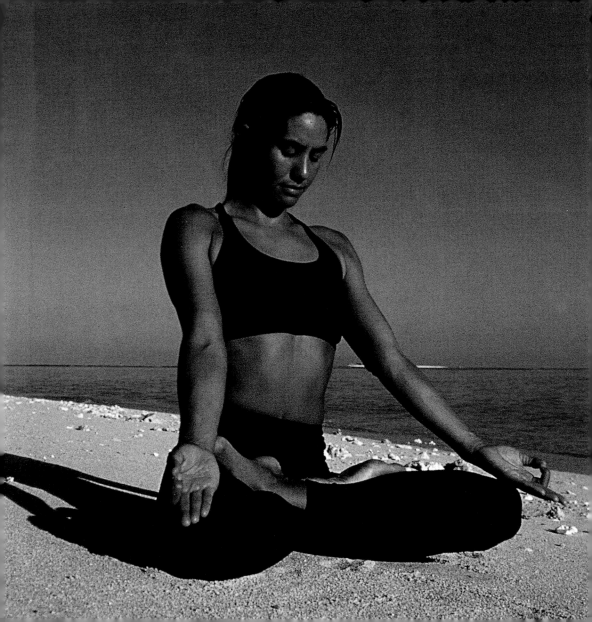

INTRODUCTION

HATHA YOGA IS FOR EVERYBODY, YOUNG AND OLD. The postures can be adapted to meet any condition or level of ability. Yoga is different from other forms of exercise in that it is not based on performance or physical strength. Yoga is not about how you look but how you feel inside. Yoga is about you being with you.

Why yoga? The key to good health lies in keeping the body, mind, and breath working together in harmony. Yoga means union of body, mind, and breath. The purpose of yoga is to calm the mind so that awareness is clear and focused. When the mind is free of worry and agitation, the body relaxes and opens. We become physically and mentally stronger.

Picture the grace of children's bodies as they dance or play. The spine of a child is supple and fluid. With age, the spine becomes more rigid. Tension hardens the joints, and muscles lose their tone. Yoga postures restore strength and flexibility. With regular yoga practice, healing and rejuvenation can occur.

Through attention to the breath, we can slow down and be more fully in the moment. This allows us to pay attention to body signals telling us we have gone far enough in a yoga posture. As a result, there is no need to push or strain. Body injuries encountered in other forms of exercise occur rarely in yoga.

Postures, or asanas, have varied effects on the physiology of the body. Backbends bring increased circulation and stimulation to the spine, improving posture. Twists invigorate sluggish organs and tissues, helping to flush out toxins through increased blood circulation. Forward bends stretch the hamstrings and back. Standing poses open the hip joints and strengthen the legs. All postures mobilize joints, making them more limber.

When we are stressed, angry, or anxious, our breath is shallow and rapid. In yoga the emphasis is on diaphragmatic breathing. A deep, slow breath brings inner calm. Through breathing exercises, relaxation, and meditation, we access greater clarity and peace—the true goal of yoga.

A BRIEF HISTORY

YOGA HAS EXISTED FOR THOUSANDS OF YEARS IN INDIA. In ancient times, practices and sacred texts were passed on orally from teacher to student. The earliest writings about yoga are the *Vedas*, ancient Sanskrit texts describing rituals and chanted hymns of devotion.

The yogic teachings are set forth in the *Yoga Sutras* of Patanjali, aphorisms or sayings about yoga written 500-200 B.C. The *Sutras* describe mental processes used to achieve clarity and connection with the Divine. The practice of yoga asanas—the physical form of yoga—is briefly noted in the *Sutras* as an adjunct to meditation.

The *Hatha Yoga Pradipika* of Swatmarama which came later describes the technique of asana practice for the first time. Over the centuries yoga has evolved into the postures known today in the West as Hatha Yoga.

The practice of yoga continues to evolve. Sri T. Krishnamacharya, who died in 1989 at the age of 101, was the predecessor of many of today's teachers, including his son, T. K. V. Desikachar, as well as B. K. S. Iyengar, Sri K. Pattabhi Jois, and Indra Devi. Each teacher has developed an individual style. Many of the studios in the West teach these forms of yoga. Hatha Yoga today consists of asana practice, breathing exercises, relaxation, and meditation techniques.

HOW TO BEGIN

WHAT DO YOU NEED TO START YOGA PRACTICE?

- an empty space or room
- a level, clean floor
- moderate room temperature with fresh air, if possible
- a firm mat, a towel, a washcloth for the eyes

- a shower to warm the muscles

- shorts, leggings, or loose fitting clothes

- undisturbed time without telephone or other interruption

Try practicing 10–20 minutes at the beginning. Work up to an hour. Set a time and stick to it, as regular practice is better than sporadic effort. You might start out practicing once a week, for example, and increase the frequency gradually.

It is useful to attend a class to have a teacher look at your alignment and form. A qualified teacher can make specific recommendations according to your age and physical condition. As with any new exercise program, it is advisable to consult with your physician first.

Select a program that works for your lifestyle and schedule. If you take on too much at once, you may not stay with it. Instead of thinking of yoga practice as a "should," think of it as nourishment for your whole being. Yoga is an investment in you.

One way to refine your ability to quiet your thoughts is through uplifting music, which settles the thinking mind in remarkable ways. Peace and clarity come quickly and easily. Try your yoga relaxation with the CD, especially if you are having trouble settling down. Let yourself float on the strains of soothing music as you unwind and let go.

Modern life is exciting and stressful. To be able to slow down, relax, and be with yourself is essential to good health. This book is a guide to a simple and safe means of caring for yourself mentally and physically. Hatha Yoga is a challenging and enjoyable way to a healthier life.

In yoga, a traditional greeting is "Namaste," accompanied by a gesture with palms together in front of the chest in prayer position. Namaste honors the light and the spirit in another. As you begin your yoga journey, we bid you, "Namaste."

YOGA POSTURES

IN HATHA YOGA, THE POSTURES OR ASANAS ARE THE CENTRAL FOCUS. Asana is a Sanskrit word which means "steady seat"—the yoga posture is held in a steady manner. The asanas emphasize joint mobility and the movement and extension of the spine.

Yoga is different from sports and other forms of exercise in that the positions are held with attention to breath and the sensations of the body. If you are off in your mind doing errands or planning dinner, you've wandered away from yoga and lost your steadiness. Yoga is awareness in the present moment. When the breath is attended to during the asana, grace and ease result.

If you are a beginner, practice the asanas in **AN EASY START** before attempting the more difficult sequence. More experienced students may do the first and continue on to the second. After gaining a sense of proficiency in the practice sequences, you will be ready for the Sun Salutation. A modified stress release program for office or airplane is included at the end.

The Sun Salutation combines many asanas into a connected flow. As the name implies, it was traditionally practiced as a way of giving homage to the morning sun that sustains all life. The Salute is a body prayer done with reverence. The fluid repetition of poses reflects the ever-changing, cyclical nature of life itself. It is both energizing and calming.

The stress release sequence can be done while seated, even in the office or in a wheelchair. Sitting for too long regardless of what you are doing causes stiffness. Over time, tension accumulates and chronic problems occur. Mental and physical fatigue take their toll. Taking time to do simple stretches will go a long way toward preventing serious injury.

Most asanas are executed to the right side and then to the left to balance the body. To start out, hold each pose for five breaths. Breathe through the nose in slow, deep breaths. Relax your abdomen. When stressed, we tend to tighten the abdomen and constrict the diaphragm. Notice any tension in your body as you hold the pose. Let your mind settle into the rhythm of your breathing. Over time, as you build strength and agility in the poses, work up to 10 deep breaths. The longer you hold, the deeper you go with your breath into the dynamic action and stretch of the pose.

Props are useful for some poses. For seated floor poses, it is important to execute forward bends from the hips and pelvis, not the lower back. If you are tight in the hamstrings or groin, sit on a folded towel. This relieves the hamstrings and allows you to come forward without collapsing over your diaphragm or straining your lower back.

Each asana addresses different aspects of the body. Note how you feel before you begin yoga practice. Choose poses that will benefit your specific needs. Because you were limber and energized yesterday does not mean that you will be today. Respect your body and energy level. Don't push too hard. Approach each asana with gentleness. Regardless of your age, 10 to 15 minutes of daily practice will be far more beneficial than occasional longer sessions.

Do not eat for several hours before you practice. Hatha Yoga cleanses toxins from the body and assists elimination. It will not work effectively if the stomach is full.

AN EASY START

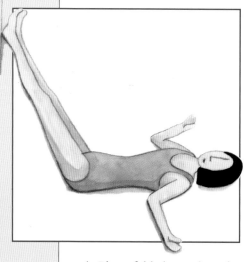

SIMPLE INVERSION

Props: wall space, towel, washcloth

Benefits: for swollen feet and ankles, varicose veins, lower back tension

1. Sit on the floor about 1 foot from the wall with knees bent parallel to the wall.
2. Pivot on your buttocks toward the wall and lie down slowly, extending your legs and placing your heels on the wall.
3. Make sure your hips are parallel to the wall.
4. Place folded towel under your head and folded wash cloth on your eyes. (Dampen cloth beforehand with cool water if weather is hot.)
5. Put arms out from the body in a relaxed position, palms up.
6. To come out, hug knees to chest. Roll to your right side and use your hands to push up.

LYING ON BACK TWIST

Prop: towel for your head

Benefits: tones digestive organs, stretches lower back

1. Lie on your back, knees bent, feet flat on the floor, arms at shoulder level.
2. Move your hips 5 inches to the left.
3. Bend your knees toward your chest.
4. On an exhalation, shift both knees and feet together to the right.
   Rest on the right outer hip, with right leg on floor. Take 5 deep breaths.
5. On an exhale, bring your knees back to center.
6. Move your hips 5 inches to the right. Repeat to the left side.
7. Come back to center.

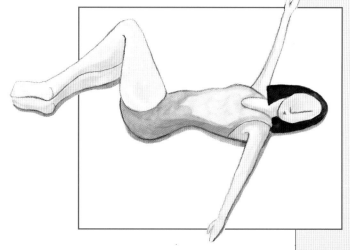

STICK POSE (DANDASANA)

Props: folded towel

Benefits: Strengthens lower back and hip flexors, extends knee joints, stretches hamstrings, tones kidneys, improves posture

1. Sit on floor, legs extended out in front at right angle to torso. Use towel as needed.
2. Place your feet together and pull toes back toward your shins to extend backs of legs.
3. Sit up on your sit bones—the bony part of the pelvis that rests on the floor.

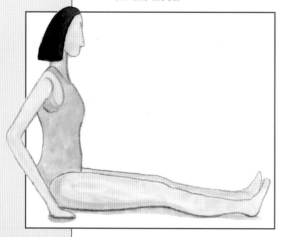

4. Place hands beside hips, bending at elbows. Use fingertips to push against floor, lifting the spine and chest.
5. Relax your abdominal muscles. Breathe deeply for 5 deep breaths.

SEATED FORWARD BEND (PASCHIMOTTANASANA)

Props: folded towel

Benefits: stretches hamstrings and lower back, extends knee joints, calms the mind

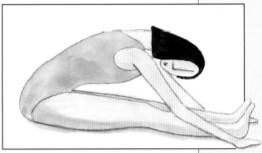

1. Sit on floor, legs extended in front, hip-width apart. Use folded towel as needed.
2. Place hands on floor behind buttocks. Press your fingertips into the floor to sit up on sit bones. Lift up your spine and lower back.
3. Push with your fingers on the floor to tilt your trunk forward.
4. Slide hands down your shins. If you are limber enough, clasp the outsides of your feet, provided you do not round the spine to do so.
5. Keep extending the front spine with each inhalation. Release into the pose with each exhalation.

CROSS-LEGGED TWIST (SUKHASANA)

Props: folded towel

Benefits: massages inner organs, revitalizes the spine, opens chest and shoulders

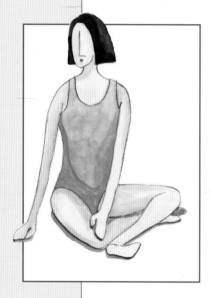

1. Sit cross-legged on floor, left leg in front. Use folded towel if needed.
2. Put right hand behind you on floor, left hand on right knee.
3. Inhale deeply and lift the spine up.
4. Exhale and twist to the right. Hold twist for 5-10 breaths.
5. Return to center. Change legs so that the right leg is in front.
6. Twist to the opposite side.

BOUND ANGLE POSE (BADDHA KONASANA)

Props: folded towel

Benefits: aids circulation to groin and sexual organs, is good for prostate, relieves intestinal congestion

1. Sit on edge of towel to lift pelvis if groin and hamstrings are tight.
2. Place soles of feet together. Let knees fall open.
3. Hold feet or ankles with your hands.
4. Inhale. Lift spine up.
5. Exhale. Relax shoulders, inner thighs, and groin.
6. Breathe and hold. Keep eyes directed toward the floor.

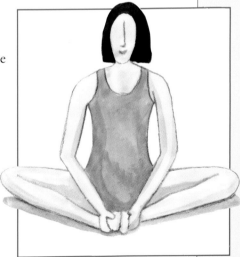

WIDE LEG FORWARD BEND
(UPAVISTHA KONASANA)

Props: folded towel

Benefits: stretches hamstrings and inner thigh muscles, works hip joints

1. Sit on edge of towel as needed.
2. Spread legs wide apart. Knees face the ceiling, toes straight up.
3. Place hands behind your buttocks. Inhale and lift spine with fingertips pressed to the floor. Open the chest.
4. Exhale and tilt forward. Slide hands down shins. Hold on to your big toes if you are limber enough.
5. Inhale. Extend front spine.
6. Exhale. Relax groin, backs of legs and abdomen.
7. Continue to extend and relax as you breathe.

WIDE LEG FORWARD BEND

MOUNTAIN POSE (TADASANA)

Benefits: enhances posture and alignment, improves balance

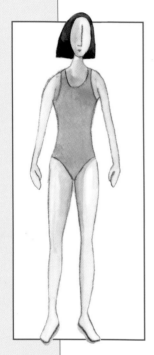

1. Stand with your feet hip-width apart. If you have difficulty with equilibrium, stand against a wall.
2. Put hands on hips and align your hips over your ankles.
3. Release your tailbone down and draw your navel toward your spine so that you are not sway-backed.
4. Lift your kneecaps by contracting the quadriceps muscles above the knees.
5. Relax shoulders and arms. Lift your chest.
6. Tuck your chin in slightly to lengthen the back of your neck.
7. Draw your attention downward to grounding of your feet and legs.
8. Let eyes gaze ahead.
9. Relax your abdomen and breathe slowly.

SWAYING PALM

Benefits: Extends spine, improves lateral flexion of spine, invigorates digestive organs

1. Stand as in Tadasana.
2. Interlace fingers in front of you.
3. Turn wrists inside out. If you have wrist difficulty such as carpal tunnel syndrome, simply clasp hands.
4. Inhale. Lift arms over head and stretch. Draw your navel toward your spine to prevent overarching.
5. Exhale. Lean to the right. Turn your chin up to the left. Hold as you breathe.
6. Inhale. Lift back to center.
7. Go to the opposite side.

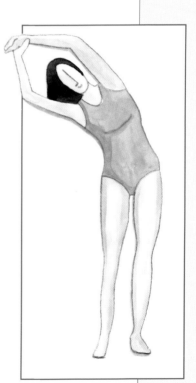

STANDING FORWARD BEND (UTTANASANA)

Benefits: stretches hamstrings, relieves stiffness of spine and general fatigue, increases blood circulation to head, improves complexion, calms the mind

1. Stand as in Tadasana.
2. Put your hands on your hips.
3. Exhale. Hinge forward at the hips.
4. Slide your hands down your legs and let them rest on your shins or on the floor.
5. Release head and neck.
6. Lift your kneecaps.
7. Relax abdomen and breathe deeply.
8. To come out, put your hands on your hips, bend knees slightly, lift your chest and press down with your feet.

RELAXATION OR CORPSE POSE (SAVASANA)

See Breathing and Relaxation, p. 42.
You may complete your practice with Savasana
or go on to the next sequence.

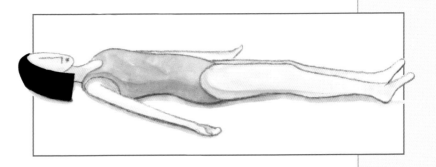

THE INTERMEDIATE SEQUENCE

FORWARD LUNGE

Benefits: stretches fronts of thighs and hip flexors

1. Start on your hands and knees (Table Position).
2. Place your right foot forward between your hands. Foot should be far enough in front so that your heel stays down with shin vertical as you lunge forward.
3. Left knee and shin remain on the floor.

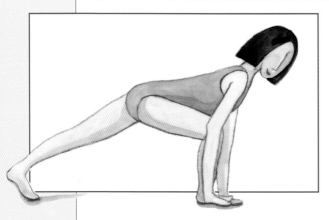

4. Come up onto your fingertips. Lift your chest up and forward. Option: To deepen stretch, curl the left toes under and lift the back knee off the floor.
5. Repeat lunge to the opposite side.

CAT TILT, DOG TILT

Benefits: teaches pelvic movement, enhances spinal flexion, coordinates movement and breath

1. Kneel in Table Position.
2. Exhale. Cat Tilt: Push with hands and arch back to the ceiling. Your tailbone draws under and your chin draws in.
3. Inhale. Dog Tilt: Chin and tailbone lift up and back becomes concave.
4. Repeat this movement with breathing three to five times.

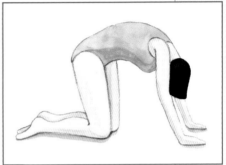

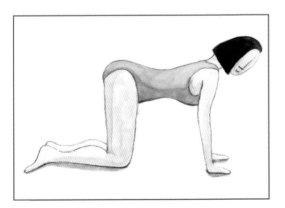

DOWNWARD FACING DOG
(ADHO MUKKHA SVANASANA)

Benefits: stretches hamstrings and calves, strengthens arms, stretches shoulders and spine, increases blood flow to head

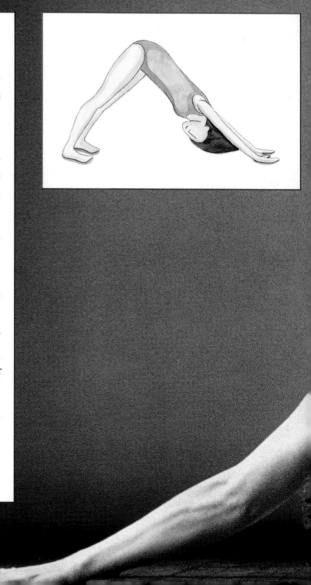

1. From Table Position (see Forward Lunge), move hands several inches forward of your shoulders. Spread fingers wide with index fingers parallel.
2. With feet about hip-width apart, curl your toes under.
3. Inhale. Lift your knees off the floor; push with your hands to extend hips away from floor.
4. As the hips and tailbone lift, lower your heels. Heels do not need to reach the floor but you should feel a calf stretch.
5. Soften your abdomen. Hold position and breathe.
6. To come out, return to hands and knees.

ADVANCED DOWNWARD
FACING DOG

(for advanced students only)

CHAIR POSE (UTKATASANA)

Benefits: stretches calves and Achilles tendons, strengthens thighs, opens diaphragm

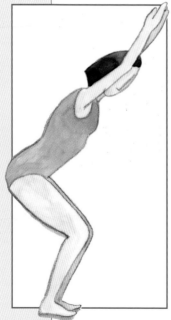

1. Stand in Tadasana, feet together.
2. Inhale. Put your palms together (namaste) in front of your chest and stretch arms overhead.
3. Exhale. Bend your knees forward over your toes. Sit back with your hips as though sitting in a chair.
4. Keep heels on the floor, weight supported equally through each foot.
5. Hold and breathe.
6. On an exhalation, straighten your legs and lower your arms.

The following three standing poses may be done with the back to the wall to enhance balance and alignment. The Standing Forward Bend, or Uttanasana, may be done between postures. Standing poses are traditionally done to the right side first, then the left.

WARRIOR POSE (VIRABHADRASANA II)

Benefits: strengthens lower legs and thighs, develops stability and stamina, helps correct knock-knees

1. Stand in Tadasana.
2. Set your feet apart (about 4 feet).
3. Stretch your arms out, palms down.
4. Turn your right foot out. Angle your left foot in.
5. Exhale. Bend your right knee to form a square over your right ankle.
6. Your chest remains vertical. Roll knees out and apart from each another.
7. Pull back with left arm. Turn your head to the right. Gaze out over your extended fingers.
8. Hold and breathe.
9. Exhale to come up. Repeat to the left side.

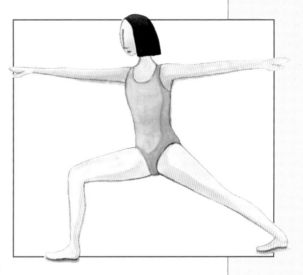

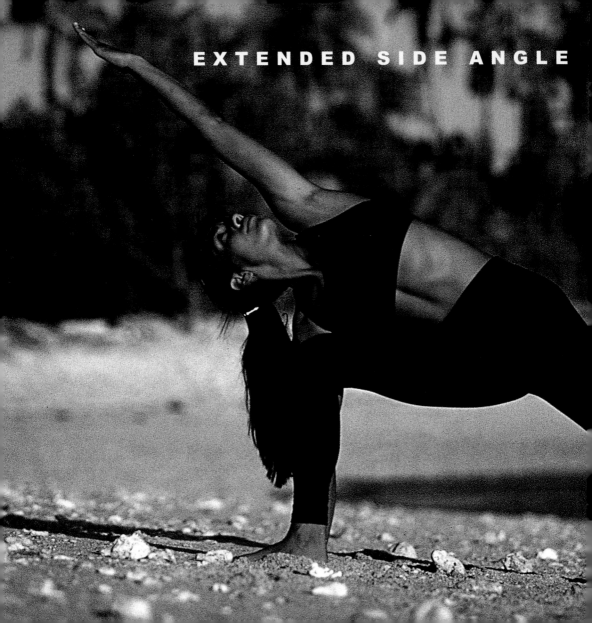

EXTENDED SIDE ANGLE

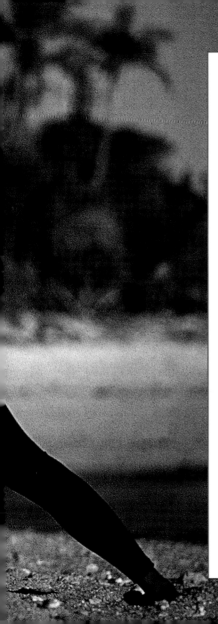

EXTENDED SIDE ANGLE (UTTHITA PARSVAKONASANA)

Benefits: stretches the waistline, strengthens and tones legs, increases flexibility in hips

1. Stand in Tadasana.
2. Set your feet wide apart (about 4 feet).
3. Turn your right foot out and your left foot in. Extend your arms to the sides.
4. On an exhalation, bend your right knee to a right angle, thigh parallel with the floor, shin vertical. The knee should be over the ankle.
5. Extend your torso to the right and place your right forearm onto your thigh. Bring right fingers to the floor behind your ankle if you want a deeper stretch.
6. Your right arm braces your right leg as you roll back your left hip and left shoulder to come into a horizontal plane.
7. Raise the arm to vertical or stretch it diagonally to the right, palm facing the floor.
8. If you feel balanced, look up under your right arm toward the ceiling. Otherwise, look straight forward.
9. Hold and breathe. Repeat on opposite side.

EXTENDED TRIANGLE (UTTHITA TRIKONASANA)

Benefits: Strengthens and tones legs, increases flexibility in hips and back, opens the groin

1. Stand in Tadasana.
2. Set your feet wide apart—about 4 feet.
3. Turn your right foot out and your left foot in. Extend your arms out to the sides, palms down.
4. Right knee cap rolls out to the right.
5. Exhale. Extend your torso sideways to the right. Place your right hand on your right leg. Stretch your left arm straight up, palm forward. Spine and head line up horizontally with your legs.
6. Hold and breathe.
7. Inhale. On the exhale, press down with your feet to come back up.
8. Repeat to opposite side.

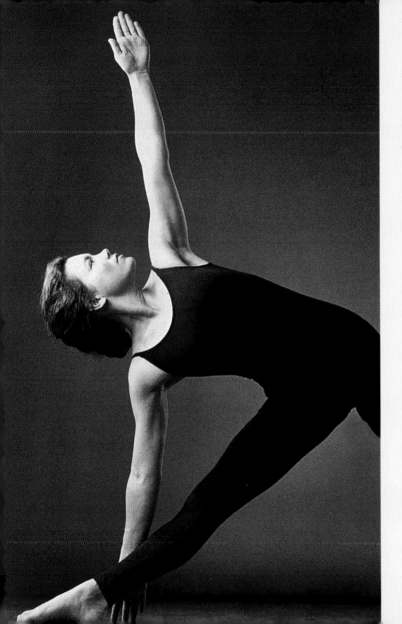

EXTENDED
TRIANGLE

FLANK STRETCH (PARSVOTTANASANA)

Benefits: stretches hamstrings, tones and strengthens legs, improves balance and stamina

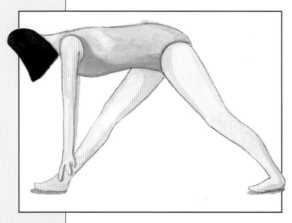

1. Stand in Tadasana.
2. Set feet 3 feet apart. Place hands on your hips.
3. Turn your right foot out and your left foot in about 60 degrees.
4. Rotate hips to face the right leg.
5. Inhale. Lift the spine.
6. Exhale. Fold forward over the right leg. Slide hands down the right leg, or along the floor on either side of your ankle if you are more limber.
7. Hold and breathe.
8. Put hands to hips. On the exhalation, press feet firmly and come up.
9. Repeat to opposite side.

BOAT POSE (PARIPURNA NAVASANA)

Benefits: strengthens front torso and thighs, strengthens back and abdominal muscles, massages intestinal area

1. Start from Dandasana or Stick Pose.
2. Draw your legs in toward your chest. Clasp your hands around the back of your knees. Lift your chest up.
3. Inhale. Lift your feet off the ground. Lean back slightly and balance on your sit bones.
4. Exhale. Straighten your legs.
5. Extend your arms out parallel to the floor.
6. Keep lifting chest as you hold and breathe.

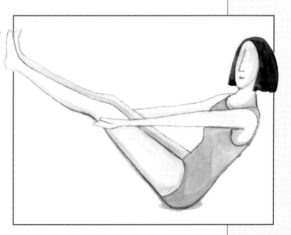

COBRA POSE (BHUJANGASANA)

Benefits: strengthens paraspinal muscles, opens chest

1. Lie down on your stomach. Place your forehead on the floor.

2. Bend your arms and place your hands on the floor next to your chest.

3. Press your tailbone down.

4. Inhale. Press your hands into the floor and lift your head and chest up.

5. Look straight ahead and breathe slowly.

6. Slowly come back down on an exhalation.

   Turn your head to one side and relax.

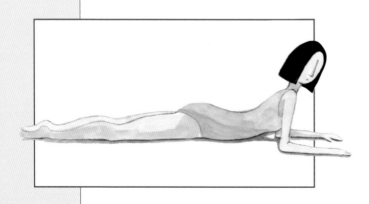

FISH POSE (MATSYASANA)

Benefits: Opens throat and chest, increases
flexibility in spine

1. Lie on your back on the floor with knees bent.
2. Slip your hands, palms down, under your buttocks.
   Keep elbows slightly bent.
3. Slide your legs out one at a time. Keep legs active by pressing backs of legs into
   the floor, keeping feet together.
4. Push down on your elbows and arch your chest.
5. Inhale. Drop your head back. Rest the top of your skull on the floor.
   Lift your sternum and chest toward the ceiling.
6. Breathe slowly and deeply.
7. To come out, tuck your chin in.
   Lie back down in a supine position.

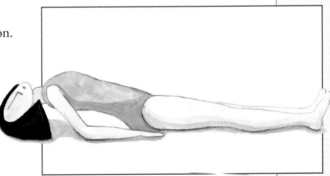

SUN SALUTATION (SURYA NAMASKAR)

Every morning, for centuries, people along the Ganges River in India have performed the Sun Salutation to greet the morning sun. One full Sun Salute cycle consists of the sequence of poses below. Do as many cycles as you wish. Experiment with pacing, moving faster or more slowly. Take time with each pose to ground yourself. Breathe deeply and move with awareness.

Benefits: Energizes and calms the mind, enhances overall toning, increases agility and flexibility

1. Stand in Tadasana, the Mountain Pose. Inhale deeply.
2. Bring hands to namaste, or prayer position. Exhale.
3. Inhale. Put arms out to side and up overhead. Look up and arch your chest.
4. Exhale. Come forward into Standing Forward Bend.

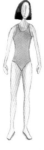 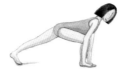 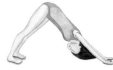 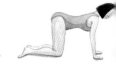

Mountain   Standing
Pose   Forward Bend   Forward Lunge   Downward Dog   Table Pose

5. Inhale. Bend your knees, bring your hands to the floor and step your right foot back into Forward Lunge.

6. Exhale. Step your left foot back into Downward Facing Dog. Take 5 deep breaths.

7. On an exhalation come onto your knees in Table Position.

8. Inhale. Move your hands forward of your shoulders on the floor.

9. Exhale. Bend your arms and glide forward onto your abdomen.

10. Inhale. Move into Cobra Pose. Take a few deep breaths.

11. Exhale. Lie back down. Place forehead on floor and inhale.

12. Exhale. Push back up to Table Pose.

13. Inhale. Step right foot forward to Forward Lunge.

14. Exhale. Step left foot forward into Standing Forward Bend.

15. Inhale. Put arms out to the side, open your chest. Slowly stand up, bringing your arms over your head.

16. Exhale. Bring your hands to namaste.

17. Begin another Sun Salutation.

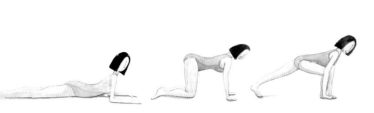

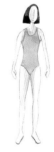

Cobra Pose   Table Pose   Forward Lunge   Standing Forward Bend   Mountain Pose

SEATED TEN-MINUTE STRESS RELEASE

This can be done easily seated in a chair in the office or on an airplane.

Preparation: Sit on the edge of your chair with spine erect. Place your feet flat on the floor, hip-width apart. Place your hands on your lower ribs and take a few deep breaths (See Breathing and Relaxation, p. 42).

1. **SHOULDER SHRUGS**. Place your hands in your lap. Inhale. Draw your shoulders up toward your ears. Exhale. Let your shoulders drop. Do this 3-5 times to release shoulder tension.

2. **ELBOW CIRCLES**. Put your fingers to your shoulders. Make a circle with your elbows by taking them forward, up, back and around. Do this 3-5 times. Reverse direction.

3. **NECK RELEASE**. With hands in your lap, drop your chin to your chest. Keep your chest lifted. Gently roll your head to the right, tipping your right ear to the right shoulder. Roll back to center and over to the left shoulder. Do this 3-5 times.

4. **FLEX AND BEND**. Clasp your hands together and cup behind your head. Inhale. Widen your elbows and arch your upper back. Exhale and draw elbows together as you drop your head to your chest. Repeat 3-5 times.

5. **SEATED SIDE BEND**. Place your right hand on the chair. Inhale. Extend left arm toward ceiling next to your ear. Exhale and bend to the right. Reverse directions, 3-5 times on each side.

6. **ANKLE AND HIP OPENER**. Sit erect on the edge of the chair. Cross the right ankle over the left thigh. Grip your left shin with your hands to maintain extension of your spine. Rotate ankle in a circle clockwise 3-5 times, then counterclockwise. Lean forward from the hips over your legs and breathe deeply for 5 deep breaths. Change sides and repeat.

7. **CHAIR TWIST**. Sit with erect spine. Put your left hand on your right thigh and your right hand on the chair next to your right hip. Inhale and lift spine. Exhale. Rotate to the right. Use your hands to help you twist. Remain in the twist for five deep breaths. Return to center and twist in the opposite direction.

8. **ALTERNATE KNEE SQUEEZE**. Sit erect. Lift your right knee up and clasp your hands around your knee. As you exhale, bring your knee toward your chest. Hold and breathe for five deep breaths. Repeat with left knee to chest.

9. **LION POSE**. Place hands palm down on your thighs. Exhale completely. Inhale deeply through your nose. As you exhale, open your mouth, stick your tongue out toward your chin. Open your eyes wide and look upward. The exhalation is a long, sustained breath. Relax and repeat several times.

10. **FORWARD BEND**. Put your feet at least a foot apart. Fold your arms onto a desk or the back of the airplane seat in front of you. Hinge at the hips. Relax and breathe. You may also fold all the way over and let your head and arms hang between your knees.

BREATHING AND RELAXATION

The purpose of deep breathing (Ujjayi Pranayama) and relaxation (Savasana) is to calm the nervous system. The "fight or flight" response is a primitive survival mechanism that activates the adrenal glands to assist you when you are in danger of being attacked. In modern life, this same adrenaline rush kicks in when you are angry or stressed. Our early ancestors could relax as soon as danger was over, but the constant demands of life today keep the adrenals in overdrive. Eventually the body breaks down. Chronic fatigue results, along with autoimmune and stress-related illnesses.

When we are stressed, our breath is restricted. In fight or flight mode, the breath is rapid and shallow. Poor posture due to fatigue or long hours slumped in front of a computer confines oxygen intake to the upper chest. Deprived of oxygen, the body and mind become sluggish.

Conscious breathing invites the mind and body to slow down. With diaphragmatic breathing exercises—which encourage a slower, deeper, fuller breath—oxygen pours into the bloodstream that feeds the inner organs and brain. Health and well being are restored.

Relaxation occurs when there is no external threat or demand. Mind and body can let go and replenish. When the senses do not have to be on alert, our awareness can turn inward to a calmer, more peaceful place. We connect with our inner selves. Within this self is a well of strength and clarity. The goal of yoga is to live from this wiser, calmer place.

BREATHING EXERCISES

To prepare for breathing exercises, choose a time when you won't be disturbed. You can do the exercises before your asana practice, or prior to Corpse Pose to enhance relaxation at the end of practice. Ujjayi Pranayama or deep breathing can also be practiced before going to bed to favor peaceful sleep.

Yogic breathing is done in and out through the nose. Air drawn in through the nostrils is cleaned and warmed before passing into the windpipe and lungs. The prana or life force in the breath can be taken in slowly like precious food.

As you exhale through the nose, you learn to regulate your diaphragm and gain control in the solar plexus. Expelling air slowly through the nose deepens the breath. This is particularly important for people with asthma or emphysema.

When breathing is shallow, it is because the exhalation is not complete. In moments of fear, the normal response is to hold onto the breath and not let go of it. Eventually this becomes a habitual response. When we exhale fully, we empty out toxins—byproducts such as carbon dioxide and lactic acid. On an emotional level, we release fear, anger, and worry. Stress flows out and away.

SIMPLE BREATHING EXERCISE WITH EMPHASIS ON LONGER EXHALATION:

Position: Lie on the floor with a towel under your head.

Lie on the floor in Corpse Pose (see p. 46). Place your hands on your lower rib cage. Close your eyes and notice how the ribs expand and contract as you inhale and exhale. Slowly deepen your breath by exhaling more fully through your nose. Prolong the exhalation. Don't push the breath out. Just allow the breath to flow out like water from a cool spring. The inhalation that follows will naturally flow in. Continue to breathe in a long, slow, steady rhythm through your nose. Do this for 5 deep exhalations; then return to normal breathing. Notice the calming effect.

BREATHING EXERCISE WITH EVEN INHALATION AND EXHALATION:

Position: Lie on the floor with a towel under your head.

With hands on your lower ribs, exhale completely. Slowly begin to deepen your breath to a count of 4 on the inhalation and 4 on the exhalation. Take your time and do not force your breath. If you feel yourself tense up as you extend the breathing, lower the count to 3. Your breath should move slowly, like clouds in the sky. As you become more comfortable with this exercise, you can increase the count of the inhale and exhale to 6 or more. If you simply allow the breath to flow deeply without effort, you will feel calm and at ease in your body and mind.

After 5 complete rounds, return to your normal breathing. Relax your arms alongside your body. Extend your legs on the floor and begin Savasana or roll to your right side with bent knees and use your hands to come up to a seated position. Move slowly so you do not jar your nerves.

Through slow breathing you can learn to slow down throughout your day. Breathing exercises open up awareness. Attention to the breath brings you into the present moment. You are no longer caught in thoughts of the past or future. Through regular practice of Ujjayi Pranayama, clarity and mindfulness are enhanced.

RELAXATION TECHNIQUE: CORPSE POSE (SAVASANA)

The purpose of Savasana is deep relaxation. The limbs, muscles, and joints go limp. The mind quiets. Like a corpse, you stop all movement and lie in stillness for a while. It is like a short nap except that you remain aware of sensations and breath.

Savasana allows the body to rejuvenate and integrate the effects of the asanas. Whether you are learning on the mental or physical level, taking time to absorb what you've learned is vital. Savasana is like a mini-vacation from the stretching and movements of asana. The body normalizes and comes into balance.

Savasana is also an exercise in letting go. The residue of mental and physical tension from your daily life disappears. Fatigue, agitation, and resistance dissolve. Resting in Savasana, if only for 5 minutes, is a critical aspect of yoga practice. It is a gift we give ourselves in order to feel more whole and centered. When we feel refreshed and clear, we carry this relaxation into all other activities in our lives.

Props: blanket to lie on, folded towel, washcloth
Option: Relax to music with the *Yoga Relaxation Music* CD.

1. Sit on the floor with knees bent. Lean back on your hands.
2. Extend your legs forward with feet slightly apart. Let your feet roll out to the sides.

3. Lie down on the floor with folded towel under your head.

4. Place the washcloth over your eyes.

5. Draw your shoulder blades and shoulders down away from your ears. Extend your arms out from your body about 30 degrees with palms up.

6. Mentally scan your entire body. Let your face, limbs and feet relax. Wherever you feel tension try to relax and let go with each exhalation.

7. Allow your attention to remain focused on the gentle rhythm of your breathing.

8. Remain in Savasana for 5-10 minutes. When your mind wanders, bring your attention back to the sensations of your body and breath without judgment. You can also notice the pause at the end of the exhalation as a means of keeping the mind present (more on this later in Meditation).

9. To come out of relaxation, bend your knees and roll to your side. Move slowly. Hurrying defeats the purpose. Use your hands to push yourself back up to a seated position.

10. Sit cross-legged for a moment. Place your hands in namaste. Appreciate yourself for the time and effort you have given to restoring balance in your life.

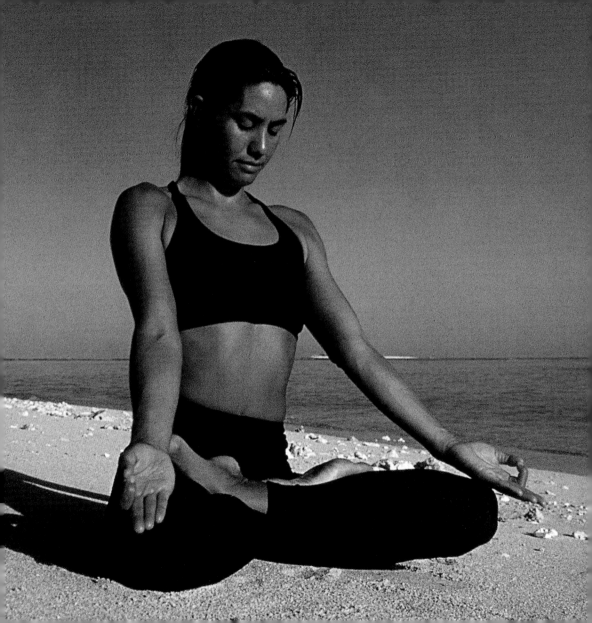

MEDITATION (DHYANA)

The desire for peace of mind is universal. No one escapes the truths of human existence. No matter how much we do to provide safety and security for ourselves and our loved ones, ultimately we are not in control of what happens. The only thing we can control is our mental attitude. Meditation is an ancient method of enhancing our capacity for serenity amidst the vagaries of life.

Joy and peace are already present within us, in our inner selves. Meditation helps to remove the obstacles of thinking that cloud the awareness of this inner self. When we learn to watch our minds, we discover a clear, calm place underneath the thoughts and emotions.

Meditation is often described as developing a witness or observer self. We watch the constant mental chatter move through us as though we were separate from it. As we strengthen our capacity to observe, we begin to see we are not our anger, our sadness, our envy, or our disappointment. We are far grander than that.

Thoughts and feelings arise out of the stories we tell ourselves about what we see occurring around us. In meditation, we notice the patterns in our interpretations. The endless stories of who did what to whom repeat themselves like television soap operas. Familiar themes and reactions replay on the screen over and over. Eventually, the stories lose their hold on us.

Meditation frees us from reaction to people and situations in our lives. The mind will always have desires, expectations, doubts, and fears. Its job is to think. Meditation is not about eliminating thought. It is learning not to identify with your thoughts. A bumper sticker says it well: Don't believe what you think.

In meditation we learn to sit quietly with ourselves and witness what is going on. As we observe the constant flow of thoughts, we come to understand that the emotional content of the mind is impermanent. Thoughts and feelings are always shifting. Anger and fear come and go. Hurt dissolves into something else. One minute we are sleepy, the next we are problem-solving or daydreaming. Everything changes. As in life, nothing in us remains constant—except our inner, observing self.

On some days meditation is easier than on others. You may find one day you are agitated or easily distracted. Other days, you settle in without effort. Training the mind to stay present is like walking a puppy on a leash. The puppy wants to stop and smell everything. You gently draw the puppy back each time and proceed on your way home.

As you develop the observer self, this detached calmness pervades all the activities of your day. You learn to identify more with the eternal you and less with the fleeting one. You will find that over time you become less judgmental of yourself and others. You can just *be* amidst the ever-changing events of your life with an acceptance of what is rather than what should be or might have been. You can be peaceful and free.

Traditionally, in India, yoga and meditation were taught from teacher to student through a lineage. The student was initiated, or given a mantra—a Sanskrit word or words charged with sacred vibration. The tone, chanted inwardly as a focus of meditation, was kept private.

There are many forms of meditation from all over the world and many books describing in detail the forms and practices. We encourage you to explore different approaches. Choose one that works for you and stay with it for a while. Be diligent. Progress will come over time.

Regardless of what method you choose, here are some basic guidelines:

- Sit comfortably in a chair or on a cushion on the floor. Your spine should remain erect throughout meditation.
- Begin with a short meditation—5 minutes is sufficient. You might feel quite restless at first. With practice, you may find you can sit longer. Add a few minutes at a time as you develop ability and focus.
- Say an invocation or prayer before you start meditation, to set your intention. Your intention might be greater clarity, inner peace, or love, for example. You might picture yourself surrounded in light or call on a teacher to help and guide you.
- Keep your eyes closed. Until you become more adept, this will minimize distraction. If you prefer to keep your eyes open, find a spot on the floor in front of you to keep your gaze steady.
- Begin your practice. Choose an object of focus (see p. 53). Each time the mind wanders from it, gently bring it back. Do not judge yourself. You are not seeking perfection, but acceptance of what is. Recall your intention in meditating.

Here are some simple examples of approaches you might want to try:

1. BREATH AWARENESS MEDITATION. The most universal focus for meditation is the breath, because it is always accessible. Bring your attention to your nostrils or your abdomen. Feel the movement of air as it is drawn in on inhalation; attend to the movement of air on exhalation. Let your breathing be normal. Watch. Let your thoughts come and go, returning to the sensation of the breath over and over.

2. **AUDITORY AWARENESS MEDITATION.** Emphasis is on the vibrational quality of sound. This could be a mantra such as "Aum" or "Ram," for instance. You could use a word such as "love" or "peace"—whatever resonates with you. The mantra or word can be said repeatedly aloud, chanted softly, or recited inwardly. Take a few moments to stop and listen to the sound. Then listen to the silence between sounds. When you find your mind wandering, come back to your mantra.

3. **VISUAL AWARENESS MEDITATION.** The focus of meditation is a visual object, like the flame of a candle or the picture of a guru, teacher, or loved one. Choose anything that inspires you—a flower, a beautiful rock. Keep your attention on the image. Keep the mind focused on the image. As soon as you find yourself drifting off in thought, return to the image.

There are many reasons why people meditate. Some want a spiritual connection to a higher power or to their inner self. Others want to be rested, better able to deal with life's demands. Some want methods of dealing with inner turmoil. Others want a larger perspective, to tap into their intuition for guidance. Once you begin to practice, you may find that meditation is essential to your peace of mind.

LIVING WITH INTEGRITY

In recent years, modern physics has proven we are all connected. Yoga teaches that our separateness is an illusion. The same molecules and atoms exist in rocks and trees, people and animals. Our survival on the planet depends on recognizing this fact.

The ancient yogis understood the interdependence of all life. The yogi of Patanjali in the *Yoga Sutras* described a system of ethical behavior to prevent inner conflict and conflict with others. The ethical code consisted of two parts: the Yamas and Niyamas. These are standards to grow toward in order to lead a harmonious life filled with grace and beauty.

The code of behavior toward others, or Yamas, includes such attitudes as truthfulness, consideration, kindness to others, moderation, and not taking what belongs to other people. The Niyamas refer to the attitudes we assume about ourselves. These include contentment with what is, surrender to a Higher Power, spiritual inquiry, and a healthy lifestyle.

There is much to be gained by reading the Yoga Sutras in their entirety. Various translations and commentaries are available at bookstores and libraries should you wish to learn more.

Yoga begins with a commitment to ourselves. Through practice of the asanas and meditation, we embark on a journey that takes us deeper into an understanding of ourselves and our connection to all of life.

On the yoga mat, we learn to be with ourselves in the present moment without judgment or comparison. Gentleness and attention to self lead to a more centered, balanced approach to others. We handle life with greater compassion and understanding. As we live in the right relationship to ourselves and others, the world becomes a more peaceful place.

Living with integrity is what yoga is all about. Enjoy the journey.

Namaste.

YOGA RELAXATION MUSIC
CD PLAYLIST

1. Kuan Yin – Troika, composed by David Arkenstone
   Published by Nara Music, Inc. (BMI)/Dream Palace Publishing (BMI)
   From the album GODDESS by Troika
   (p) 1996 Music Design, Inc.

2. Crystal Fantasy, composed by Michel Genest
   Published by Nara Music, Inc. (BMI)
   From the album CRYSTAL FANTASY
   (p) 1984 Sonia Gaia Productions

3. Wind and Willow, composed by Wayne Gratz
   Published by Nara Music, Inc. (BMI)
   From the album PANORAMA
   (p) 1990 Narada Productions, Inc.

4. Quiet Heart, composed by Richard Warner
   Published by Nara Music, Inc. (BMI)/Quiet Heart Music (BMI)
   From the album QUIET HEART, SPIRIT WIND
   (p) 1996 Narada Productions, Inc.

5. Inner Flame, composed by Richard Warner
   Published by Nara Music, Inc. (BMI)/Quiet Heart Music (BMI)
   From the album QUIET HEART, SPIRIT WIND
   (p) 1996 Narada Productions, Inc.

6. Going Home, composed by Wayne Gratz, Nancy Rumbel
   Published by Nara Music, Inc.
   From the album REMINISCENCE
   (p) 1989 Narada Productions, Inc.

Narada has become one of the world leaders in defining and establishing new instrumental, jazz and world music, always evolving, diversifying, and setting new trends. Narada is home for many exceptional recording artists who are creating cutting edge music today.